EMOTIC
THR
BREAST CANCER:

THE ALTERNATIVE HANDBOOK

DR CORDELIA GALGUT

In loving memory of my mother, Sheila

12-10-30 to 13-3-11

Radcliffe Publishing Ltd
33–41 Dallington Street
London
EC1V 0BB
United Kingdon

www.radcliffehealth.com

British Library Cataloguing in Publication Data

A catalogue record for this book is available from the British Library.

ISBN: 978 1 84619 936 3

Typeset and designed by Moo Creative (Luton)
Cover designed by Tracey Thomas
Printed and bound by CMP (uk) Limited

WHAT PEOPLE SAY ABOUT THIS BOOK

'The truth of what it is really like to experience cancer is laid bare in this book. The voices of so many women expose the reality of how cancer affects every cell in your body and every facet of your life. Cordelia's humanity, understanding and empathy with cancer patients/sufferers shines through every page. Despite the pain expressed by so many women this book is full of hope. Cordelia's understanding, her explanations of how people might be feeling, her practical suggestions on dealing with common issues, her clarity and compassion, all make this a book that will support every woman with a breast cancer diagnosis, no matter how recent or how long ago. The truth on every page of this book is unlike any other book or material I had read about cancer. For the first time I realised that the way breast cancer had affected me was not unique. I was not crazy or even abnormal to feel the way I did. I did not have to be ok and feel lucky because I had survived. It was not weird that once the treatments had finished that everything did not fall into place. It was not unusual that I felt let down by the system or by some of the medical staff or by some of my family or by some of my friends. Breast cancer and going through breast cancer treatment are profoundly disturbing experiences for many people and the impact of going through these is profound and lasting. Above all Cordelia's book shows how this is and why this is. It should be available to every woman, to every friend, to everyone who cares. And it should be compulsory reading for every health professional who comes in contact with cancer patients.'

Rosa Lopez
Diagnosed 2012

'Cordelia brings a very special perspective to the experience of breast cancer – both professional and personal. Without frightening women, she is honest about the challenge of treatment and, for me, more importantly, the mental battle to face life post cancer.'

Louise Davies
Diagnosed in 2011

'Tells the unspoken truth about what having breast cancer is really like.'

Lindsay Nicholson
Editor, Good Housekeeping

'As an oncologist, I know that the emotional impact of breast cancer is often devastating and Cordelia does not shy away from this. This book will help you to understand your emotions and cope with them.'

Dr Carmel Coulter
Consultant Clinical Oncologist

'I urge everyone who has been diagnosed with breast cancer – or who wants to understand what to say or do to help someone they know – to read this book. Cordelia Galgut includes perceptive insights into the life-changing emotional impact of this frightening diagnosis and outlines strategies for supporting yourself or a loved one through the experience. It's eleven years since my own first-hand experience and this book's suggestions are hugely helpful and relevant to me still.'

Joy Ogden
Medical journalist and author of Understanding breast cancer, (John Wiley)

'Being both a woman who has experienced the trauma of living with breast cancer and also being a healthcare professional, I feel this book reflects both sides of the coin with great truthfulness and clarity. It was helpful to me to finally read a no holds barred account of what women really feel, especially once their treatment is over and life is often expected to 'get back to normal' when this is definitely not the case. Dr Galgut brings together her own experiences plus that of many other women to show that the impact of breast cancer on a woman's life is often something that continues long after diagnosis and treatment.'

Sarah Cordery
Healthcare professional
Diagnosed 2010

'This book reflects the reality that living with cancer is crap and it's okay to feel that way. It's a refreshing change from the nauseating positivity of all those sky-diving, marathon-running cancer survivors we usually hear about.'

Anne Dean
Healthcare professional
Diagnosed in 2001

'This manual won't provide all the answers, but it will make sense of your feelings, thoughts and emotions. Whatever stage you're at dealing with breast cancer, this manual offers support and understanding covering not only you but those close around you. Written by Dr Cordelia Galgut, a professional and someone who has personal experience, this manual is an honest account of the realism of dealing with breast cancer. Having been diagnosed five years ago, reading this manual helped me to realise that I'm not on my own.'

Johanna Coady

'In a chapter of the book Sick Doctors, published in 1973, written by an anonymous doctor, herself a breast cancer patient, the author said, "it is important that someone with sufficient psychological insight and ability to handle the patient's depression and anger should be available in times of crisis." Cordelia Galgut, a doctor of psychology, in this support manual, provides such an insight as well as sympathy and empathy, which is also necessary as part of understanding. As a retired general medical practitioner whose wife developed breast cancer, I now know better than most how terrifying breast cancer is. Still today, in 2013, the psychological impact of breast cancer is worse than the disease itself, which can be effectively treated today, in most cases.

I therefore recommend this manual and consider that it would be useful reading for doctors, nurses, patients and, for that matter, anyone who meets and cares for breast cancer patients.'

Dr Iain Esslemont
Retired GP

'A unique perspective of the psychological effects of breast cancer.'

Catherine Stubbs
Healthcare professional

CONTENTS

CONTENTS

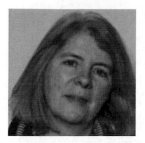

About the author

Dr Cordelia Galgut is a practising BPS Chartered psychologist, an HCPC Registered counselling psychologist and a Registered MBACP senior accredited counsellor/psychotherapist. She is widely published on various aspects of psychology, counselling and psychotherapy, and since her breast cancer diagnosis in 2004 has often written about the emotional impact of breast cancer from her dual perspective as psychologist and breast cancer sufferer. Her book, *The Psychological Impact of Breast Cancer*, was published by Radcliffe in 2010.

Acknowledgements

I am indebted to Liz Lane, for her unequivocal support of my writing and this project. Words cannot express my gratitude.

Many thanks also to those at Radcliffe/Speechmark who have been involved in this project, especially to Tanya Dean and Anne Renton for their unstinting commitment and hard work.

An enormous thank you to Dr Deirdre King for her extremely useful contributions.

I am also indebted to the following for their invaluable help and support with this book:

Isabel Bristowe
Johanna Coady
Sarah Cordery
Dr Carmel Coulter
Dr Iain Esslemont
Mary Esslemont
Michael Galgut
Catherine Hadjiminas
Dr Caroline Hoffman
Louise Johnston
Ruth McCurry
Dame Jenni Murray
Lindsay Nicholson
Joy Ogden
Maeve Ryan
Anne Shewring

A huge thank you to Kate Condliffe for carrying out the arduous task of typing and re-typing drafts of the book and for her unerring support throughout.

Last, but by no means least, a huge thank you to all those of you whose testimonies enormously enhance this book. Without your words, it would have been considerably less meaningful, so I thank you all from the bottom of my heart for your crucial contributions.

Photographs of the author by kind permission of Macmillan Cancer Support.

Introduction

The shock of being diagnosed with breast cancer is hard to describe in words, as anyone who has had to suffer this diagnosis knows. Until it happens to you, you cannot really know how it feels. Not only do we have to deal with the diagnosis and subsequent treatments, but we also have to deal with the fact that breast cancer profoundly affects how we feel about ourselves as women.

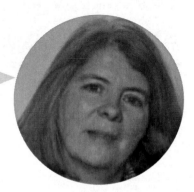

I know this because I am a counselling psychologist who has also had breast cancer. I was diagnosed with bilateral breast cancer nine years ago, at the age of 49, so I do understand first hand what it's like to find out you have this disease, and what it's like to live with it over time.

For many of us it is the hardest thing we have ever had to deal with – not least because it is our lives that are threatened and because, for many of us, its emotional and physical effects persist. **Fortunately, most of us live for years after a diagnosis of breast cancer these days**, including women with a secondary diagnosis, but it is hard to hang on to and believe this fact, even many years after diagnosis.

Why I have written this book

I have written this book to offer you:

- a different perspective from the usual one on breast cancer's emotional effects

- some emotional support

- some practical suggestions that can help you to take charge emotionally.

About this book

- If you have just been diagnosed, you might want to start with the *Just diagnosed* section (page 60). Depending on how you're feeling at this time, you may then want to read more of this book, perhaps dipping into some parts and skipping others. Equally, you may want to put reading the rest on hold for a while.

- I hope that my dual perspective as a psychologist and as a woman who has had breast cancer will offer you support that is particularly valuable to you. What I say or suggest is based on what I have learnt while coping with primary breast cancer myself, as well as from my psychological training and professional experience. It is also based on things many other women have told me.

- I hope this book helps you, whether you have just been diagnosed, are in the middle of treatment, or are a year or two beyond the original treatments or several years or more on from diagnosis. No matter what stage you are at, some parts of this book might be more relevant to you, and/or appropriate for you, than others. You might identify with some parts and not others. However, what holds true for breast cancer – that there is no right way to 'do' breast cancer – is also true for how you use this book: there is no right way!

- Also, I know that not all of us struggle with everything I raise in this book, and I want to make it clear that I believe that all our experiences are valid, whether they are in line with what you read in this book or not. Even if they are not, I hope you find its content interesting.

- This is not an advice manual. Anything I say in this book is just a suggestion or idea – I cannot guarantee that it will be helpful to you, although I hope it will be. Only you can decide how to think and feel about breast cancer, and I do not believe that anyone, including me, has the right to tell you otherwise.

- Please bear in mind that the exercises in this book may not be helpful if you are feeling acutely distressed. If this is the case, it could well be more beneficial for you to talk to a trained practitioner face to face.

- As I have no personal experience of secondary breast cancer, there are bound to be omissions, for which I apologise. However, I hope that much of what I say in this book will be of relevance to women with a secondary diagnosis. Equally, a male sufferer might well identify with some of what I have included in this manual, but again there will be omissions.

Moving on

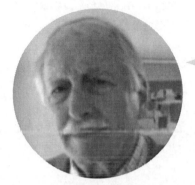

We often hear talk of how we need to 'move on' and 'get over' breast cancer and be positive. Many of us report getting heartily fed up with hearing such advice. Being on the receiving end of these judgements can make breast cancer much harder to deal with than it already is, because we then feel under pressure to achieve unrealistic goals, and then feel bad about ourselves when we can't manage this. In addition, you may have noticed that a lot of the books, leaflets and websites at our disposal tend to talk in these terms as well. They also tend to focus on the impact of cancer generally, rather than specifically on the effects of breast cancer.

Sarah says:

I've been in remission for 3 years now and often still have people saying to me that 'I should be happy now' and 'I've been given a new lease of life' so I should 'get out there and enjoy every day of it'. It's hard for people to realise that I'm still adjusting to not only the physical changes to my body but also the enormity of the whole situation I've been through. I don't want to jump out of an aeroplane or see the Great Wall of China, I just want to learn how to be the 'new me'.

Louise, diagnosed 2 years ago, says:

My body has not been the same since my treatment. Not only did I have chemo and massive surgery (double mastectomy with reconstruction), I also went into menopause as a result of my treatment (I'm 47). I have lots of aches and odd feelings and these really stress me. I find I get into a spiral of physically feeling bad which then leads to depression. I worry about plaguing the oncologist or my GP with these concerns. For example, I have backache, about which my oncologist says she is not worried, but which I find difficult to come to terms with. Some days I feel like the only thing in my head has been concerns about my health. It's like a great weight in my head. I am then split between trying to find answers – why does my back hurt? – which will involve further tests and medical visits, in themselves stressful, or just getting on with things and accepting that this is the new reality. I tell myself that I could cope with the latter if I knew for sure that it wasn't cancer, but not sure what it would take to really convince me.

Like Sarah and Louise, you might well have realised that it is not so easy to 'move on' or 'get over' breast cancer, much as we might long to. Indeed, there are many obstacles that prevent us from doing so that people in all walks of life often don't understand. However, as a woman who has had two diagnoses of breast cancer, I do understand.

What affects how we feel through breast cancer?

Our experience of breast cancer is affected by a number of factors that we all experience, but that we may not be consciously aware of at diagnosis or in the days and months afterwards. Nevertheless, the following factors inevitably affect, to a greater or lesser extent, the way that we think and feel about our situation, and can make coping with this illness and 'moving on' even harder.

It can help and support us to realise that these factors exist and can impact negatively on us as we cope with breast cancer.

Prognosis

Obviously, the way that we feel is affected by how advanced our cancer is and the type of cancer that we have. If the cancer has spread beyond our breasts, we will experience extreme doubts and fears about our future. If we have early stage breast cancer, we are also very likely to have extreme doubts and fears for our lives. However, there is clearly a difference between having a primary and a secondary diagnosis, although with the latest medical treatments women can live for many years after a secondary diagnosis. In fact, these days, breast cancer is being viewed increasingly as a chronic illness that can be controlled, rather than as a fatal disease.

Treatment

Our experience of breast cancer will also be affected by the kinds of treatment we have for it and how we cope physically with that treatment. Some of our systems will cope better with the treatments than others, whether we have a primary or a secondary diagnosis although most women will not find them a breeze, either psychologically or physically. Recognising that you are not alone in finding the treatments difficult can be very reassuring – many women have told me it is a relief to find out that their reactions are normal.

A major reason why we can end up feeling as though we are not reacting normally is that we are often told that everyone reacts differently to the various treatments. Certainly, it is true that we are all individuals and some of us will indeed find them easier to cope with than others, either physically, psychologically or both. However, many of us have reported similar reactions. For example, even though we know that we are having treatment for our own good, we can feel very vulnerable and even violated after surgery and during chemotherapy and radiotherapy.

This view is confirmed by Dame Jenni Murray, who said of her experience of chemotherapy:

> *It runs counter to any principle of self-preservation.*[1]

This reaction is common enough, but is seldom talked about and not well understood, and it often helps women to know that they are not alone in feeling like this. It can also be a shock to learn that treatments go on for so long. The public perception of treatment for breast cancer is that it is over fairly quickly, whereas, as we know, it usually goes on and on, in a way that is totally exhausting. I want to reassure you that you are not alone if you feel or have ever felt like this.

Myths about treatment

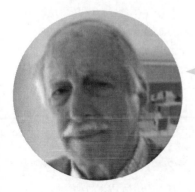

> MYTH:
> These days, chemotherapy
> and radiotherapy are easy
> treatments to cope with.

Sarah, diagnosed 3 years ago, says:

Not enough preparation and warning is given to patients about not only the immediate effects, but also the long-term effects I'm still feeling now. I felt I wasn't prepared enough for my radiotherapy treatment, it was almost glossed over and expected to be 'a walk in the park' compared to the 8 sessions of chemo I had just undergone. When taking into account how weak your body and mind are from the treatment you have just finished, the radiotherapy is then everyday. I found it exhausting just getting to and from my appointments, but mentally and emotionally I was reminded about my illness every day. For 28 days, my life consisted of nothing but cancer, machines and doctors – it didn't seem such a walk in the park!

Magda says:

The treatments were not easy, but I felt better physically than I expected to. It was the emotional effects that got me. They hit me out of the blue. Nobody had told me I'd feel so at the mercy of the machinery and the people organising the treatments, and I still haven't got over that.

Lou says:

I was diagnosed with breast cancer in May 2001, and had surgery followed by a course of chemotherapy and radiotherapy. The chemotherapy made me feel pretty awful, tired, drained of all energy, but I was prepared for that and admit it wasn't as bad as I thought it would be. I was less prepared for how bad the radiotherapy sessions made me feel. I had to drive about 45 minutes every afternoon for the treatment, and sometimes struggled to get home again. After the sessions I would feel dizzy, my legs would feel as if they wouldn't hold me up and I felt nauseous. You don't generally hear that radiotherapy will make you feel ill, and feel that it should be a breeze, but I would say it was almost as hard to get through as the chemo.[2]

Rosa says:

I wish that someone had talked to me about the treatment in advance, that someone had explained exactly what would happen, what position I would have to lie in, how the radiotherapists would have to concentrate all their attention on ensuring that the position was correct and would have no time to be concerned about the emotional impact on me, and especially if someone had to!d me of the feelings that could arise for me. I

> *know now that not everyone experiences radiotherapy as such a brutal and traumatic treatment. But it would have made such a difference if someone had told me that I might feel disempowered, exposed, controlled, violated, victimised. Because that is how it felt, but for a long time I thought I was the only person in the world who had ever felt this way because of this treatment. I thought I was going crazy. If only someone had prepared me, if only someone had told this truth.*

As Sarah, Magda, Lou and Rosa have all said, treatments are made harder for us if we are not told what they can really be like. The harshness of them can then come as a total shock, whereas those of us who have been prepared well can sometimes find a treatment easier than we feared, as Lou pointed out. Also, some aspects of the treatments are not even familiar to many of our doctors and nurses – for example, the fact that they can make us feel so vulnerable. People outside the medical and nursing professions are often even more ignorant of or can turn a blind eye to their real effects – both physical and emotional. As you have probably noticed, many people, including some health professionals, tend to assume that:

- treatments are easier to cope with than they often are

- they are over and done with quickly

- the emotional effects of the treatments are seldom significant.

As women coping with this diagnosis that is so desperately hard to deal with, we can end up feeling even more miserable, confused and torn because of the ignorance of others and their unwillingness to accept this reality.

As a result we can then easily feel that we are not coping with breast cancer 'properly' if we find the treatments too hard or are too upset and depressed during or after them. We can feel as if our reactions are not normal, even though they are. It can then be hard to admit, either to ourselves or to others, how we really feel.

As a psychologist, I want to reassure you that:

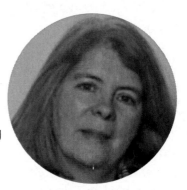

- The deep emotions that we feel ongoingly, to varying degrees, after a diagnosis of breast cancer, and during and after surgery, chemotherapy and radiotherapy, are normal.

- Most women find the different treatments hard to cope with. Some of us find one treatment more difficult to cope with than another, and some of us struggle more emotionally than physically, or vice versa. Sometimes we feel under pressure to say that we are fine and/or that the treatments are fine both during and after the initial treatments have ended. However, most of the women I have spoken to since I was diagnosed admit that:

  - they struggle, to a greater or lesser extent, to cope with the side effects of chemotherapy, radiotherapy and hormonal treatments

  - they censor what they tell people, including family, friends, doctors and nurses, for fear that they will be judged 'too anxious', 'not coping' or 'going mad', and because they don't want to offend or upset anyone. For example, Suky commented that 'Everyone's inevitable lack of awareness made me very angry and very upset, all of which was kept inside as we are not supposed to make a fuss, are we?'[3]

Photograph by kind permission of Macmillan Cancer Support

- Extreme, deep and long-lasting emotions are a perfectly normal reaction to breast cancer diagnosis and its treatments – not least of all because breast cancer can recur and the effects of treatment can endure. Although we know that women can live for years after a secondary diagnosis, a recurrence or spread of the disease is not what any woman with a primary diagnosis would want, and feeling terrified of this is perfectly normal and to be expected.

- Depression, although very unpleasant, is a very common and normal response at any stage during breast cancer, even long after all the treatments are over.

Enduring emotions

Sarah, who was diagnosed three years ago, said:

The fear of cancer returning is something you never get used to. I get irritable, angry and at times often irrational when it comes close to my 3-month check-up. It's not even something I consciously put myself through, it's just always there in the back of my mind.

You might well be able to identify with the way that Sarah feels, and also with the following statements:

- It is hard, if not impossible, not to be terrified of recurrence, and this fear and terror does not go away, even if we shove it down as much as possible. It's always there, just beneath the surface.

- For a significant number of us, the fear of recurrence can get worse over time. If it does, this is perfectly understandable, not least because the longer we live post-diagnosis, the more we dare to believe that we will survive breast cancer. Many of us also fear having to have more treatment.

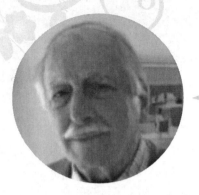

MYTH:
You should be over breast
cancer by now – it's not
normal.

- We all fear that we will lose our lives to breast cancer, even if we can barely admit this to ourselves, let alone to other people.

- We can easily struggle to 'move on.' This is perfectly normal, and there is no set date by which any woman diagnosed with breast cancer should feel she has to 'move on.' It takes time to adjust to this diagnosis, and the whole concept of 'moving on' is often unhelpful, as it puts us under pressure that we could do without.

- As human beings, most of us will deny how we are feeling even to ourselves at some point, some of us more than others. This is perfectly normal. It is not pleasant feeling miserable, and denial can be a coping strategy as well as a shock response. Also, as human beings, we are often not conscious of what is going on for us under the surface. Each one of us has a lot going on, on an unconscious level, that we are not aware of, but that might nevertheless affect us. For example, we might feel very irritable or angry out of the blue. This is perfectly normal, albeit unpleasant.

Perhaps you will also recognise some of your own reactions in the following description of Tash's situation.

Tash was diagnosed with breast cancer in her left breast two years ago. It was a small cancer, so she had breast-conserving surgery.

Nevertheless, she has two long scars – one on her breast and one under her arm. Since there was some lymph node involvement, she had to have chemotherapy. She also had four weeks of radiotherapy to her breast. Since then she has been on Tamoxifen. She says:

People tell me I should be over breast cancer by now and, in a way, I think I should, too. I mean, it's two years now. My husband has been great, but even he is losing patience with me now. The trouble is I don't feel right at all. I hide my feelings from him, from my children, my friends and my colleagues, and to be honest, I'm not sure how I feel sometimes and I shove things down myself because I've got enough on my plate as it is. I know what I have been through has been really rough on me and I'm screaming inside, and I also don't feel as well as I did before breast cancer, but I also put pressure on myself to feel okay and can't easily talk about how I feel. I lie awake at night panicking and wondering if the cancer has spread and if my number is up, and this Tamoxifen is driving me crazy. It makes me feel so ill and emotional. I tell myself it's helping to keep the cancer away, but in the middle of the night it's hard to remind myself of that. Why can't I just get over everything? I mean, I'm okay, at least I think I am. My scans are okay and nobody is telling me I'm not.

Here is my reaction, as a psychologist, to what Tash says

Obviously, Tash's situation cancer-wise is only one version of breast cancer. Some women have a better prognosis than Tash and some have a worse one, and some women have had a diagnosis of secondary breast cancer. Some women will be suffering less than Tash and some will be suffering even more than her. However, one of the many things we all share, apart from the fear we will die of this disease, is that we all have to cope with other people's reactions to us. We also have to cope with our own conditioned responses. For example, like Tash, many of us have a voice inside our head telling us that we shouldn't feel too upset or too scared through breast cancer, and of course it doesn't help that this message often comes across loud and clear from the people around us.

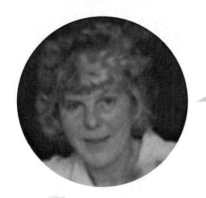

MYTH:
It's not normal to
be so upset.

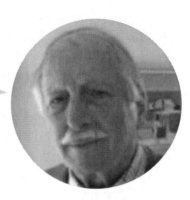

TRUTH:
Breast cancer is a
profoundly upsetting
experience.

Some practical suggestions that might be helpful

It doesn't help if, on top of suffering from the fallout of breast cancer, we end up censoring our own thoughts and feelings because we believe it is wrong to have them. **There is no right way to 'do' breast cancer. Furthermore, by giving ourselves a hard time for feeling what we are feeling, we might well be making things harder for ourselves**. It is fine if we genuinely feel positive about our situation. However, if we are putting ourselves under pressure to feel positive because we've been told that this is the right way to be, and we are bottling up our real feelings, this will add to our stress levels. We may worry that if we don't stay positive, our cancer will return, because this is a common belief that we will inevitably pick up on. **However, there is evidence that maintaining a positive attitude makes no difference to whether our cancer will return or not**.[4]

Repeating affirming sentences
There is some evidence that if we repeat affirming thoughts and feelings to ourselves over and over again, we can change our thought processes from unhelpful ones to ones that are more supportive of us.

Here are some affirming sentences that you might like to try. Choose one or more of the following that appeal to you, or make up your own version if something that is more relevant to you springs to mind. Repeat the sentence over and over out loud.

- I'm doing really well getting through this.

- I'm allowed to feel as bad as I like.

- I'm allowed to feel angry and upset about what's happened to me.

- I'm allowed to feel okay.

- There's no right way to get through breast cancer.

- I'm allowed to feel positive.

- I'm allowed to feel depressed.

- I'm allowed to say 'no.'

- I'm allowed to feel terrified.

- I'm allowed to feel sick to death of everything.

- I'm allowed to get angry with people.

- I'm allowed to feel lousy.

If you feel like changing what you're saying to something else, mid-repetition, that's fine. Sometimes the phrase that you choose will gain momentum, so you might start with 'I'm very angry about what breast cancer has done to me' and feel like changing it to 'and I get furious when people tell me to get on with it and be more positive.' Swearing is good for expressing the strength of your feelings, if you're okay with that; try to avoid muting your feelings by saying 'quite' when you really mean 'very.' If you're very angry, say that you are very angry or furious. Doing these affirmations might make you feel more angry and upset and maybe scared. This is a perfectly natural way to feel and react. Stop if it gets too much for you. If it helps, your last affirmation could be something like:

- We **do** survive breast cancer these days.

Some people find that writing whatever they want on Post-It notes and sticking them around their home in key places is useful. Because these notes give visual as well as verbal reinforcement, this can help to support us, too. Others make affirmation cards. I certainly know of women who, during their treatment, when they were too exhausted to do much else, spent time making cards for themselves and found decorating them quite therapeutic as well. Some women use them to communicate their feelings to the people around them, too, when they are too weary to explain how they feel. They're not always very polite, but they make us feel better! Most of us have some days that are better than others. Overall, though, these women say it's good to know it's normal and okay to have plenty of negative thoughts, too!

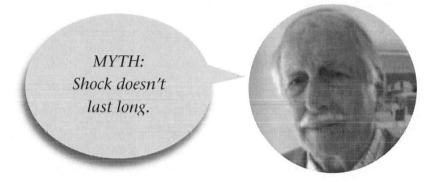

MYTH:
Shock doesn't
last long.

Longer-term shock

Although most of us will recognise that we are in shock at diagnosis (see the *Just diagnosed* section on page 60), we may not realise that shock endures. It can help and support us to realise this, as it takes some of the pressure off us to feel okay when we know we don't feel that way. It is perfectly normal to be in shock for months and even years after a major life trauma, and breast cancer is clearly one of these! We seldom speak about shock as anything other than an emotion that is transient – a short-lived thing. In reality, this is not so. The trouble is that there is little public awareness of what a shock response actually is for us as human beings. We will, of course, be in shock at diagnosis– stunned shock, numb shock. That is a given, but Suky's version, which is described below, is common, too.

Suky says:

> *Living with trauma does not become easier over time – in fact it becomes a more isolating experience as the general assumption is that as time has passed, one should be over it. My diagnosis, operation, chemotherapy and radiotherapy experience happened six years ago, and whilst I am able to 'forget' for significant periods of time, it doesn't take much to bring back the overwhelming sense of fear and panic, a reaction deemed by everyone, except those I know who have gone through the same diagnosis, to be over-reacting.[5]*

As time goes by and we move through to life beyond the initial treatments, we will often be far less aware of how shock is impacting on us. We could easily be post traumatically stressed, as well, a large part of which is a shock response. The trouble is that most of us have had not one shock (diagnosis) but multiple shocks to our system, caused by surgery, chemotherapy, radiotherapy and hormonal treatments. Each shock can easily make the others harder to cope with both at the time and afterwards as well. To explain - when, as human beings, we experience multiple shocks to our system and psyche, as we do through breast cancer, our systems get overloaded. It's easy for us to feel frightened and/or terrified a lot of the time and 'on alert', waiting for the next horrendous thing to happen, even years after diagnosis. The fact that the memories endure does not help. And, of course, for most of us there are constant reminders – for example, our scars, on-going pain and the fear that our cancer will return or get worse.

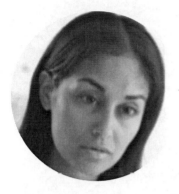

TRUTH:
The effects of the first
shock can make the second
one harder to cope with,
and so on.

So shock can get layered on top of shock, even if we find our treatments relatively easy to cope with. We can easily still be in shock from our diagnosis and then shocked again by all of the things that we have to endure as part of having breast cancer. Each shock can make the following one even harder to cope with, because our systems are so weighed down and overloaded by all that has happened and is happening. This is inevitable, but is seldom understood, even by our doctors and nurses.

It's hard for those supporting us, namely oncologists, nurses and other health care professionals, to really take on the reality of how we feel unless they have been through breast cancer themselves - they are seldom trained in depth in the psychological impact of breast cancer. Furthermore, their jobs are hard ones and in order to help them to cope, a normal protective response for them is to cut out awareness of how the treatments are affecting us, as patients. This doesn't help us emotionally, but it allows them to do their jobs without getting too distressed.

Sometimes shock can be delayed, as in Melanie's case, when it seemed to come from nowhere.

Melanie, diagnosed two years ago, says:

> *I actually found the treatments I had okay at the time. They were hard, but I coped with them fine, emotionally. Recently, I've been having weird flashbacks and often feeling a bit panicky. I'm not sure why, but I didn't expect to feel like this now and it's quite scary.*

Melanie is having a delayed shock reaction. This is not unusual and is perfectly normal. Although she hasn't been consciously aware of how she has been feeling about her diagnosis, she has been processing what's happened to her and not forgetting it. For example, her fears for her future haven't gone away. It takes time to adjust to a different version of ourselves. The rug has been pulled out from under Melanie's feet. Although time will help her get more used to her changed situation, she will never be quite the same again – not necessarily in a negative way! Again, it might help her to keep reminding herself that she is allowed to feel what she feels, now that she has become consciously aware of her panicky feelings.

There is also some evidence that relaxation exercises which shut down our fight or flight response, that makes us feel wound up, frightened and anxious, are useful. Melanie might be able to learn to control her panic, without pushing it away, by trying the following exercises, as might any of us if we are feeling like Melanie.

Switching off your fight or flight response

Dr Deirdre King, an autogenic therapist, suggests that the following body scan may be helpful:

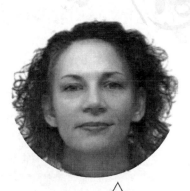

Ongoing stress keeps the fight–flight response switched on for long periods, causing a further stress. Relaxing switches on the rest–recuperate response, which allows your body to repair itself. If you feel comfortable connecting to your body, you could try this body scan. Find a quiet place where you will not be disturbed. You might like to shake surface tension out of your body first and take a couple of deep breaths. Sit or lie comfortably and close your eyes. Then take your attention to your body and gently scan either up or down it for a few minutes. Notice how you feel and any physical sensations, the pulses and rhythms of your body. No need to try and change what you observe. Accept it, without judgement or criticism, as what is going on for you right now. Let your breathing do what it does naturally as you quietly observe. At the end of your body scan, yawn, stretch and open your eyes; get up slowly.

If emotions come up, try to acknowledge them and let them be. You could try the offloading exercise described on page 31 to relate to your emotions, but leave an hour before or after doing a body scan.

The longer-term impact of trauma

The stages through which we are supposed to progress after an extreme shock are not, in reality, what happens. Popular culture suggests, and indeed medical and mental health professionals have often been taught, that after a major trauma such as a diagnosis of breast cancer, we should expect to go through a process of emotional recovery that lasts for a set period of time. At first we are shocked, then we go into denial about having breast cancer, then we get angry, then depressed, then finally after a year or so we accept what has happened to us and move on.

Bola says:

> *I feel tons better for realising I don't need to go through all the different stages. I couldn't understand why I wasn't feeling loads better a year after I was diagnosed. I'm a doctor, and the medical view tends to be that there's something wrong mentally if you don't respond a certain way after trauma. I now recognise that these models are unrealistic and I feel relieved. I feel what I like, when I like, knowing this is entirely normal.*

The trouble with this model of trauma response is that we are expected to go through stages in a linear fashion and 'get over' the trauma. The problem is that this is not how we naturally react as human beings. For example, it is totally possible to experience shock, anger and depression at the same time, or not to connect with these emotions at all. And the problem with breast cancer is that we can never really get over it, so long as the fear of recurrence and death is there and so long as the scars remain and the effects of treatment continue.

- Perhaps the best way to cope with these ongoing fears is to recognise that they are normal and that our task is to learn to live alongside them, as best we can, and remind ourselves that some days will be easier than others.

- Talking to people about our fears can help some of us. Somehow, daring to speak them to someone can be a relief. Others of us will not want to surface this fear and terror any more than is necessary, and that is fine, too.

Why can people, including those of us with breast cancer, often act as if breast cancer is easier to live with than it is?

This is a complex question, but there are some clear explanations, too.

- Within Western society, and the UK is no exception, we tend to make light of the emotional impact of traumatic experiences on us. Most of us have been brought up to believe that to dwell on suffering is an indulgence, and we shouldn't do it. This sets up a conflict in us, including those of us with breast cancer (as I often see in my consulting room). We know that what we are going through is appallingly hard to bear, but we've been conditioned to make light of it.

- Furthermore, people around us can expect us to be over the treatments and back to normal fast, because this is easier for them to cope with.

- As a result, family, friends, colleagues and the health professionals supporting us, most of whom will have been brought up similarly, will tend to collude in the myth that awful traumas in our lives are easier to cope with than they are.

Rosa's family and friends' reactions bemused and upset her.

I didn't know what I expected from my friends and family members. But once I started radiotherapy treatment I felt absolutely on my own, and let down by everybody. People who didn't contact me at all. People who contacted me and didn't understand. People who made vague offers of help 'if there was anything they could do.' People who asked me how I was but obviously wanted me to say I was fine. People who said how important it was to keep 'positive.'

Not everyone will react like this, but when people do, these might be some of the reasons why they respond in this way.

- Those around us are understandably very frightened of cancer/breast cancer and of dying and serious illness generally. It is perhaps easier for them emotionally to turn a blind eye to our suffering. That way, they don't have to dwell so much on the things that scare them.

- Those of us who are affected by the disease can react similarly. Perhaps we should feel less frightened, given that these days even women who have had a secondary diagnosis can live for years. However, as I know full well, that's easier to say than do. Of course, those of us living with a breast cancer diagnosis want to control this fear and terror as much as possible, too, but it is generally harder for us to do so than for those who are unaffected.

Amy says:

I was diagnosed ten years ago now. Even so, I fear those annual check-ups as much as ever – more than I used to, actually. It shocks me that I do. You'd think I'd be more optimistic now I've survived for ten years. It's confusing and nobody understands how I feel, and I suppose I feel silly really. Other women who've had breast cancer say the same thing as me, though, thank goodness, that it gets harder over time. I guess I'm terrified it'll come back and I don't want more treatment, I don't think I could bear that.

- Furthermore, because of our conditioning, it is generally hard for us to tolerate our extreme and enduring emotions. As children, many of us were trained to try to control our feelings. The classic example is that of the child who falls over, who is naturally in pain and upset, but is told to ignore it and 'get on with it.' Or the child whose grandparent dies and who is told not to dwell on their sadness. This sets up a situation psychologically where the child starts to feel that their reaction is not normal if they feel intense and/or protracted grief, although this is a normal reaction to being bereaved, or to coping with any kind of extreme trauma – for example, breast cancer!

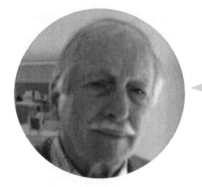

MYTH
You shouldn't be
sad anymore.

- Therefore many of us have not been taught how to cope with our own extreme and enduring emotional responses, other than to try and keep a lid on them. When we find ourselves, in this case, diagnosed with breast cancer, it is easy for us to get very scared of our extreme emotional reactions to what is happening to us, even though they are perfectly normal. We can easily start to feel that we are going mad, even though we're not, we're just having a normal, human reaction to being in such a horrible situation.

- The reality is that, as human beings, we are wired to have extreme and enduring responses to things that happen to us in life. When our own lives are threatened, we are bound to have very extreme emotional responses, not least of all terror. Why wouldn't we?

Practical tips

It can help if we allow ourselves to validate our emotions. For example:

- It's completely normal for me to feel so terrified and out of control. I'm not going mad.

- I don't have to keep a lid on my feelings if I don't want to. They're just a normal response to what I'm going through.

- It's okay to keep a lid on my feelings if I need to, but I know my feelings are totally normal.

Intentional offloading exercise

Dr Deirdre King, autogenic therapist, says:

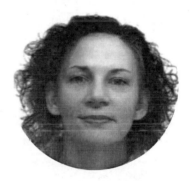

If you do want to release feelings that you think have got stuck, you could try the following: This exercise, based on an Intentional Offloading Exercise from autogenic therapy, helps to release feelings that have got 'stuck.' It is not necessary to actually feel the feelings whilst you do this exercise, although it's fine if you do.

First decide what you want to work on – for instance, you could work on your sense of shock and panic. Find a place where you will not be interrupted to do your exercise. It is best not to do it an hour or so before going to bed or doing a relaxation exercise or meditation. Always work within your comfort zone, stopping if you feel uncomfortable.

Take a single phrase that strongly expresses how you feel. Repeat the phrase out loud over and over again until you come to a natural stop or the phrase becomes mumbling. For instance, you might say 'I'm scared' or 'I'm scared of dying.'

Pause to check if you need to repeat it some more or if any other phrase comes up. If so, continue as before. New phrases may come up quite naturally. Work each through to the end until no new phrases come up and you feel calmer. Try not to stop too early, as this can leave you feeling anxious, irritable or headachy, but do stop if it gets too much for you. If it feels right, you can also use body movements to express how you feel, like wringing your hands or pacing.

This exercise usually takes between 5–15 minutes.

Relationships

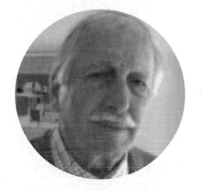

MYTH:
Relationships don't
change as a result
of breast cancer.

Relationships of all kinds are hard, as I know well, not just from personal experience, but also from all of the people whom I have supported professionally with their relationship issues over the years. Any kind of trauma, including breast cancer, can easily put a strain on even the best relationships. However, as adult human beings, most of us seldom say how we feel – most of us have been taught not to! This sets up a situation whereby there are huge unspoken agendas between us all – things we think and feel, but don't say. During times of trauma, these agendas can get even longer and more heartfelt. In an ideal world, perhaps we would talk openly about how we feel. However, the reality is that each one of us may not necessarily be consciously aware of our unspoken agendas in their entirety, only of parts of them. Also, many of us will probably not have the energy to try to sort out these problems during breast cancer. Sometimes, perhaps the best way to cope is to acknowledge that there are differences of opinion between you and people in your personal life or between you and those in charge of your care, and leave it at that for the time being. Sometimes, though, it will be important to say things to help yourself feel better.

Do you recognise any of the following 'unspoken' thoughts and feelings, either about partners, family, friends and colleagues or about the medical professionals who are looking after you? If you do, you are not alone! Many of us feel like this often enough. I certainly do.

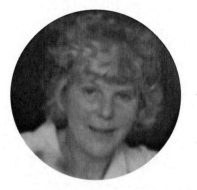

> *TRUTH:*
> *Unspoken agendas*
> *are normal – we all*
> *have them.*

Family and friends

Sophie, who was diagnosed with breast cancer four years ago, often thinks the following about some of her family and friends, but hasn't spoken her thoughts to the people concerned. Other women have said they think similar things:

- 'I feel so alone. They haven't got a clue what I'm going through.'

- 'I know they're trying to help, telling me how to think and feel, but if they were in my shoes I don't think they'd be much different, whether they talked about how they were feeling or not.'

- 'They make me angry.'

- 'I'm sick to death of breast cancer and all the problems it's caused me.'

- 'I'm still terrified it's going to come back. I feel as though all I get is a limited reprieve between my check ups, though any little signs or symptoms during those periods still send me into a panic. They don't understand this. I've tried to tell them how I feel, but it hasn't changed how they are with me.'

- 'My life has changed so much, but they don't get that. They expect me to get back to normal now, but I can't, and I never will in the way they want me to.'

- 'I can't when I'm reminded every day of breast cancer when I see my scars and have pain in my arm and back and have to take my pills.'

- 'I want them to feel better about me, but I'm struggling myself. I haven't got the energy to help them out right now.'

- 'I wish they'd just leave me alone for a bit.'

- 'If somebody tells me to be more positive again I'm going to scream.'

The following are some unspoken thoughts of Sophie's partner, Jim, and some family and friends:

- 'Why does she go on about how she's feeling? Can't she keep it to herself? She's driving me insane. Why can't she be more positive? It was ages ago now.'

- 'She shouldn't be talking like this. It's not good for her and it makes me feel uncomfortable. I'm sick to death of breast cancer.'

- 'I'm frightened of getting cancer and dying, and her talking about it is making me more frightened.'

- 'I'm still frightened she'll die. I want her to be okay.'

- 'I want to help, but I don't know how to. Everything I try to do seems wrong.'

- 'I need a break. She makes me angry.'

- 'I don't really understand what she's going through. And I don't really want to. It's too hard.'

- 'I want everything to go back to normal. Why can't she just get over it and get back to how she was? She's okay now, her cancer has gone – she's being unreasonable and making things worse for herself and me.'

In the case of Sophie and Jim, they decided to go to a relationship counselling service where they were offered a few sessions for free. Not everyone wants to involve a professional in their personal problems; also, not everybody can afford to pay for this kind of help if it is not available free of charge. However, Sophie and Jim did find it helpful.

After their six sessions were over, they both agreed that having a trained professional in the room with them, listening to them both and summing up what each of them was saying and putting it to the other person, was really helpful. At home, they would just get into arguments and not listen to each other.

Jim said:

> *It was really useful that the counsellor suggested each of us spoke for a few minutes about how we felt, without the other one interrupting. I knew I had to be quiet and not interrupt, and I think I really heard how Sophie felt for the first time since she was diagnosed. The counsellor then suggested I repeat what she'd said, as in saying to Sophie that I had heard what she said and listing the things she'd mentioned. She really appreciated that, and I felt like we'd communicated properly for the first time since she was diagnosed. She also listened to me saying how I felt. I'm not ashamed to say I cried. I've felt so alone and distant from her, and the counselling has brought us together again.*

Sophie said:

> *It's been great being able to say all the no-go things in a safe environment. I knew the counsellor would jump in and redirect and contain us if things got out of hand, and that's been really helpful. I definitely feel I've got a lot off my chest. I understand Jim's position better, and we've got strategies for helping us cope, which is really great. I wish we'd done the counselling sooner.*

Strategies for helping us to communicate with family and friends

Here is an exercise you can try with anyone in your personal life that might help communication between you (even work colleagues, if they agree). You could even try it with your younger children, aged about seven plus, if the strategies are adapted and turned into a kind of game. The strategies in the exercise are similar to the ones Sophie and Jim learnt about, but they're not just for partners. They take a bit of getting used to, and might feel strange at first, but there is plenty of evidence that exercises such as this one can aid communication between people, and very few of us find that easy!

You'll need a stop-watch or something similar for these exercises.

- Suggest that you and the person in question sit down facing one another somewhere comfortable.

- Tell the other person that you would really appreciate them listening to you for two minutes, without interrupting, and then tell them whatever you want to, e.g. 'I hate it when you tell me I should be over breast cancer by now. I can't be because ...'. It's better to set an alarm so that they won't clock watch rather than listen to you!

- Invite your partner/friend/family member/work colleague to say how they feel for two minutes, without you interrupting them.

- When each of you has said your piece, do the same thing again, but this time use your two minutes to sum up what you remember of what the other person has said to you. Even if they feel misunderstood, the person who is listening must not interrupt.

- Take two minutes each again and tell one another what you think of each other's summary. It's very important to do this without judgement. Is it accurate? If it is, say so and thank them for listening and understanding. If it isn't, tell them why it isn't, e.g. 'I didn't actually say I'd over-reacted to breast cancer – I said I've had a strong reaction, and to me that's very different'.

- Take a further two minutes to tell one another what you like your partner/friend saying to you and what is not okay, e.g. 'I really like it when you tell me you understand how I feel. I hate it when you tell me I'm over-reacting'.

- Finally, give one another two minutes to say what each of you has learnt about the other from this exercise.

You can adapt this exercise to suit you better. The main thing is to help you and your friends, family, partners and work colleagues to communicate more easily.

Relationships with doctors and nurses

Doctors and nurses are often grateful if we are able to be honest with them about how we feel. Unless they have been through breast cancer themselves, they cannot really know how we feel, so a major way that they can find out the reality is through us. Some will be more receptive than others. Some doctors and nurses will also be grateful if you are clear with them about what you need from them. This is easier said than done when dealing with a diagnosis of breast cancer, but it's worth thinking about trying to do so, if you're up to it.

As Louise says:

Talking to medical staff is really key, even if it's hard.

If you're not happy about something, do consider trying to talk to the people in charge of your care, as there might well be things they can do to help. If you don't feel like saying something yourself, you could ask someone else to do it on your behalf. If you're happy with what your doctors and nurses are doing, it might be a good idea to say so too, and positive feedback does seem to aid communication!

Sally's experience with her oncologist was positive:

She was in the middle of radiotherapy and summoned up the courage to tell her oncologist that she felt really upset and vulnerable lying on the radiotherapy table, and was extremely relieved when her oncologist took on board what she'd said and asked the radiographers to cover her up as much as possible during treatment, so that she was not lying completely bare-chested on the table. She was really pleased she'd asked, as she'd almost bottled out of coming for treatment because she'd felt so exposed and upset. The rest of the treatment was then much easier for her to cope with emotionally.

Don't forget that breast care nurses are there for you and they are used to helping women at diagnosis and during the initial treatment phase. Some will be more forthcoming than others, but their job is to support you emotionally as well as clinically. They do not have training in counselling skills, but they do have some training in communication and emotional support skills, so it is always worth approaching a breast care nurse at your hospital or clinic – they might well be of help to you.

Less positive experiences

Unfortunately, significant numbers of us have come across a doctor or nurse who is not as helpful or receptive as we might need them to be, and this can be very upsetting, especially when we feel vulnerable and scared.

A considerable number of women have told me they have felt variations on the following about a doctor or nurse, and felt powerless to do anything to improve the situation for themselves with the doctor or nurse in question. However, it has been helpful to them to realise that they are not alone in feeling the way they do.

These women have thought:

- 'I wish they had more time. This person is too preoccupied to attend to me as I'd like. They have to see far too many patients.'

- 'They're comparing my situation to X and Y and wondering why I'm making such a fuss. I'm glad I'm not X or Y, but I'm sick of being dismissed because my prognosis is good and I've survived for several years. My situation is still hard to cope with and there are no guarantees.'

- 'They don't recognise how stressed their job is making them. I wonder if they're looking after themselves enough.'

- 'They still don't seem to have much idea of how breast cancer continues to affect me psychologically, or physically, come to that, and worse still they're too quick to judge. I'm sure they mean well, but I'm sick of their trite comments.'

- 'I'm frightened to tell them how I feel, in case it affects my care, and I don't think they'd get it anyway.'

With the health professionals who are not so receptive

It can help if we at least recognise and try to accept that:

- they genuinely don't understand how we're feeling
- they've probably got too much on their plates
- their hands might be tied
- they're only human
- they probably want to do the best for us, but they are just not trained to understand our emotional responses.

We can then be more realistic in our expectations, which might, in turn, enable us to get more of what we need from them clinically, if not emotionally.

Remember that there will also be doctors and nurses who are thinking the following:

- 'I wish she'd tell me how she really feels.'

- 'I don't want to ask in case I upset her even more.'

- 'I don't think I'm doing my best for her, but I want to.'

- 'I'm not sure what she needs from me.'

As a last resort, remember that you have a right to change your doctor or nurse if you are unhappy with them. This can be a hard thing to do, but is always possible and you would not be the first person to have done so! However, it is for you – and no one else – to decide whether or not you need to do this.

Getting emotional support through breast cancer

Many of us, including psychologists like me, need emotional support through breast cancer, and find such support invaluable. One good thing about getting support from a trained professional is that you don't have to worry about what you say to them. They are used to hearing about a vast range of experiences. They are also not part of your life, and you can speak to them about anything in confidence and expect not to be judged. Some of us are lucky enough to be offered some counselling as an adjunct to our treatments, or get such support quickly through our GP. Some pay for emotional support, and others cannot afford such a luxury.

Whilst there is no substitute for a good, face-to-face relationship with a counsellor, I have included in this book much of what I, as a counselling psychologist, would offer a woman going through breast cancer. What I cannot offer you in this book is the personal contact and closeness of a one-to-one, face-to-face, therapeutic relationship with a caring professional (and, of course, I do not have knowledge of your personal circumstances and needs). And there is no denying that women with breast cancer often find a face-to-face relationship particularly supportive, especially when the counsellor understands them well.

Unfortunately, as with doctors and nurses, not all mental health professionals will understand our situation, much as they might try to and want to. Good counsellors will admit when they don't understand, and move heaven and earth to try to do so. A good counsellor will also know his or her limitations and suggest someone else who might understand our situation better. You have a complete right to ask a potential therapist what experience they have with breast cancer and whether they have personal experience of it. Some will be happier than others to answer these questions, but how they respond will in itself give you an indication of whether this person is the right counsellor for you or not. Leila and Resa had somewhat different experiences with their counsellors.

Leila really liked her counselling sessions:

I found the sessions I had with Mollie really helpful. She told me straight away she hadn't had breast cancer, which I really liked as there was no pussy-footing around the subject. She also said she'd had a couple of friends who'd been diagnosed, and was very real with me about the shock I felt. The main thing I liked was she was just another woman in the room, sitting with me, listening, doing her best to understand and not judging me. It was great.

Resa didn't find her counsellor very helpful:

> *Ruma was really nice, but she just didn't understand. She couldn't cope with the idea of breast cancer either. I could see her fidgeting and looking really awkward, as though she wanted the session over. She kept telling me to be positive and do relaxation exercises, so I didn't go back!*

Louise said of her experience of counselling:

> *Both during and since my treatment I have spent money on a counsellor, which was and is definitely worthwhile. Sometimes it was just 50 minutes during which I could cry without anyone in my family knowing.*

If you are seeing someone through your GP or hospital, they should have, at the very least, a basic level of qualification (e.g. a diploma in the field). You have the right to check the qualifications of the person whom you are entrusting with your psychological care, whether you are seeing them on the NHS or privately. This can be done either by asking them directly or/and by checking on the following UK professional associations' websites:

- the British Association for Behavioural and Cognitive Psychotherapies (BABCP)

- the British Association for Counselling and Psychotherapy (BACP)

- the British Psychological Society (BPS)

- the Health and Care Professions Council (HCPC)

- the Professional Standards Authority for Health and Social Care (PSA)

- the United Kingdom Council for Psychotherapy (UKCP).

Is this fear of cancer/breast cancer made worse by anything else?

The answer to this question is yes. Most of us have been brought up to believe that cancer usually kills, and tragically it still does. However, **most of us survive cancer these days**. Nevertheless, the fact that cancer is still often referred to in hushed tones, as the 'C' word, speaks volumes about how most of us think and feel about it, as the disease that dare not speak its name. Indeed, there is still plenty to fear. However, as a society we perhaps make things worse for ourselves by often still portraying cancer as exclusively a killer. Tragically, significant numbers of people do die of cancer, but the majority live on.

With breast cancer, the good news is that treatments have massively improved survival rates. However, those of us diagnosed with this disease have to live thereafter in the knowledge that either it has returned or could return at any time. This is something people often don't understand. They'll say, 'Well, you've got the "all clear" now, haven't you?' My response these days is always 'Nobody will say that anymore. Yes, as each year goes by, it seems that my chances of a recurrence probably diminish, but that's all anyone will ever say.'

Louise, who was diagnosed two years ago, says:

When people ask me how I am, I still can only say something like 'Fine, touch wood.' I use terms like 'touch wood' or 'fingers crossed.'

All cancers are hard to live with, but is there anything about breast cancer that is different?

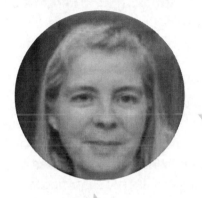

TRUTH:
The bad press that breast cancer has had for centuries affects how we feel about it today, even though survival rates have improved so much.

TRUTH:
Breast cancer has a 3000-year recorded history of failed attempts to cure it.

Yes, breast cancer has the longest recorded history of any cancer – 3000 years. During this time there have been many failed attempts to cure and treat it. As the breast is accessible, all sorts of lotions and potions have been tried on it, with the aim of curing breast cancer. Few of them have worked, and this fear of breast cancer being always a killer has therefore been passed down through the generations for centuries, so that even in the late 1950s and 1960s in England, when I was growing up, that was the prevailing belief. And of course many more women did die of breast cancer then – maybe not as many as I might have thought, but the legacy of it always being a killer prevailed. **In the last two or three decades, survival rates for breast cancer have rocketed, and treatments are much**

more effective. However, few of us have caught up with that fact in our heads, because most of us were conditioned in our youth to think about breast cancer as a death sentence. Also, it's hard to forget what a serious illness breast cancer is, because the treatments are still so extreme, there are often long-term effects and the disease can recur.

Symbolism of the breast in Western countries

Within our society, women's breasts are associated not only with sex and eroticism, but also with fertility, childbirth and breastfeeding. Most of us don't consciously walk around thinking about our breasts in this way and can be very shocked by how much this diagnosis strikes at the heart of who we are as women. However, it's not surprising that it would, horrible though it is to feel like this, when we consider how the majority of us were brought up to view our breasts. Whether we have well-proportioned ones that look good is pretty important to the average woman and remains so throughout her life, even after a diagnosis of breast cancer.

As Dame Joan Bakewell confirms:

> *What is clear is that breasts matter more to us than, say, bunions or warts, or even hip joints and rheumatism. The other conditions may be painful, but they don't strike at the core of women in quite the same way!*[6]

The way that breasts are talked about by many men in our culture doesn't help, and as women we can collude in this version, too. Most of us view women's breasts as less attractive as they age, and increasingly women have plastic surgery to make their breasts look younger. These views are unlikely to help a woman going through breast cancer. Breasts are also meant to be smooth and unblemished, and it's hard, if not impossible, to go through breast cancer treatment and emerge with such breasts, even if we had perfect breasts beforehand. Most of us would claim that our breasts do not define who we are as women, but for most of us it is nonetheless hard to feel as attractive with damaged breasts. It is a rare woman who comes out the other side of breast cancer treatment thinking that she has better-looking breasts than she did beforehand. Some women genuinely do, but they are in a small minority.

Imogen says:

I wasn't a great fan of my breasts before breast cancer. They were just there, really. My girlfriend liked them more than I did, and still does. I wonder how she'd feel if it were her in my position. I'm really shocked that having them cut into and the skin damaged by radiotherapy has made such a difference to how I feel about myself, but it really has. I still can't quite fathom why, but I'm less confident sexually than I was, and I feel less of a woman. I hate feeling like this and it makes me feel angry that I do, but I just can't shift how I feel, even though it was seven years ago that I was diagnosed. I'm not sure I ever will. Perhaps if I stopped worrying about how I feel I'd feel better. I know other women feel the same way. A friend of mine has the exact same situation with her boyfriend. He's great and loving in bed and tells her she's beautiful all the time, but she feels like I do and she was diagnosed nine years ago now.

Practical tip

It can help us to start to think of breast cancer as a chronic condition, both physically and emotionally. Not all of us will want to view breast cancer like this, and not all of us will feel like Imogen, but for those of us who do, it can help us to recognise and try to accept that the problems we are left with will be chronic ones. This takes the pressure off us to 'get over them and move on!' Strangely, it can then be easier to live with this diagnosis and its effects as the years go by.

As Louise says:

> *I find thinking of breast cancer as a chronic condition really helpful in accepting that my body has changed as a result of treatment and that these changes continue to have an effect on how I feel.*

Why can having breast cancer make us feel bad about ourselves?

Almost every woman with breast cancer will be likely to struggle to feel good about herself, at some stage, after this diagnosis. These feelings are often much more far-reaching than negative thoughts and feelings about our physical appearance alone. I have certainly struggled in this area and still do, and I have spoken to many other breast cancer sufferers who feel the same way.

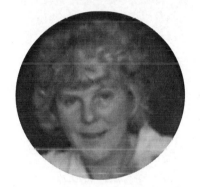

TRUTH
It's normal for our self-esteem and self-confidence to be scarred by breast cancer.

Melodie's story is much like those of many other women I have talked to over the last nine years. Perhaps you can identify with some aspects of it. Melodie was diagnosed five years ago:

When I was diagnosed, I just wanted the cancer out of me. I didn't really care at the time how that happened, except that I knew I didn't want a mastectomy unless I had to have one. It didn't occur to me that I'd have problems with the way I looked afterwards. Nobody pointed out to me at the time that even if you have breast-conserving surgery, you're usually left with big scars. I really don't have the confidence I used to have in the way I look.

> *I've felt much more vulnerable since diagnosis and treatment, and that feeling hasn't gone away, unfortunately. At least I know it's not just me, because I go on the Internet forums sometimes and other women say the same thing. In the bedroom, it's not great these days. I can't move like I used to and certain positions are really painful. I'm also pretty menopausal and get really sore, so full-blown sex is the last thing I need right now. I prefer being cuddled, but my partner wants sex so I do it, but I seem to have lost the will. Sometimes it's more pleasurable than others, especially when we stop short of penetration, and he tries his best to work round my problems, but I have to be feeling better about myself than I do to enjoy lovemaking. I wish he could see my problems as a problem shared, but he doesn't really. He just doesn't seem to get it when I tell him that I don't feel good about the way I look. He tells me he loves me and the way I look, but I'm not totally convinced and we never really talk about these things. I think we need to, but I don't know how to and I know he gets upset, too, and doesn't really understand what's going on for me. To be honest, I don't either a lot of the time. I mean, why should breast cancer make me feel this bad?*

Why can we easily feel this bad?

This is a complex question, but in a nutshell:

- An assault on our breasts is an assault on our sense of ourselves as women. Despite improvements in breast cancer treatments, they are still an assault, even though nobody planning and administering the treatment would want that for us.

- Treatment for breast cancer is inevitably invasive and leaves scars, often both physical and mental ones. It is easy for us to feel very vulnerable and exposed during treatment, and to remain so afterwards. We have to adjust to different ways of being, and few women will say they are unchanged after a diagnosis of breast cancer. Not least of all, we have to adjust to a changed body and changed life situation – our life is now threatened in a way that it wasn't for most of us before, even if our prognosis is good.

- The hormonal treatments often make us feel physically unwell, and it can be hard to carry on as normal. It's easy to lose confidence in our body's ability to work properly, and this can affect how confident and relaxed we feel in all situations, including the most intimate ones.

- It doesn't help that the hormonal treatments for breast cancer make a lot of us age faster and invariably catapult many of us into an artificial menopause.

- Younger women often have to cope with losing their fertility before having or completing their families, and even if women don't want children or any more children, the loss of the ability to have a child can make a woman feel old, bereft and 'on the shelf.' As we know, society's view of older women is not very validating of us as we age, and most of us try our best to stay young-looking for as long as possible, for fear of becoming 'invisible' women who are no longer sexually attractive. Even for a strong woman, who questions these oppressive ways of thinking about women as they age, it is hard not to be affected by others' attitudes towards us, and breast cancer just makes the physical ageing process even more challenging.

Am I to blame?

Feeling in any way responsible for our own breast cancer doesn't help us feel good about ourselves, either. A lot of us beat ourselves up to a greater or lesser extent about what we have and haven't done to cause our cancer. And, of course, we are constantly bombarded by people in the medical community and the media telling us what we should and shouldn't be doing to avoid breast cancer. Irritatingly, the reality is that many of us led healthy lives and were, for example, considerably thinner at diagnosis than we are now, after all the treatment.

Many of the hundreds of women I have spoken to since being diagnosed myself feel incensed that this culture of blame exists in our society. Having breast cancer is hard enough, without being held to task for what we have or haven't done. Having breast cancer is punishment enough, and the reality is that despite the many advances there have been in our understanding of what causes breast cancer to develop and in ways to manage the disease, as yet **no one knows with absolute certainty what causes breast cancer**. There are many recognised risk factors, but this does not mean that, if we had them, they definitely caused our original cancer, or that if we still have them, we will develop more cancer. As we know, there are many women who have risk factors and who do not develop this disease. However, it can be hard to hold on to these facts in the face of others' attitudes. Although often well meaning, they can make us feel even more miserable, if we let them.

Practical tip
It can help us to remind ourselves and other people that nobody knows definitively what causes breast cancer.

It might also help to try an exercise based on Emotional Freedom Technique (EFT). Exercises such as these can help us to feel calmer and more accepting of ourselves and our situation.

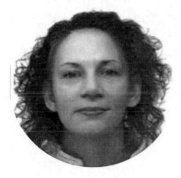

Dr Deirdre King, an EFT practitioner, says:

You could try using an affirmation which acknowledges conflicting feelings whilst tapping on a meridian point to help clear blocked energy to calm yourself. To do this you need to tap gently with two or three fingers on the fleshy side of your hand between the base of your little finger and the wrist (the part of your hand that you would use to do a karate chop).

At the same time, repeat your affirmation out loud, at least three times. Use words that really reflect how you feel. For example:

- *Even though I feel damaged and unattractive, nevertheless I can still accept myself and love myself deeply.*

- *Even though I worry that I am to blame for getting cancer, nevertheless I can let myself off the hook and still love myself completely.*

Long-term effects of treatment

For significant numbers of us, even many years after diagnosis, we suffer the emotional and physical aftermath of treatment. This is seldom understood, recognised and accepted by either medical people or the world at large, which makes coping with these long-term effects harder. Fortunately, the climate in the UK seems to be changing a little, for example Macmillan Cancer Support's publication, *Cured – but at what cost?*[7]

Ruby's situation is common:

It's seven years ago now since I had my treatments. I was on Tamoxifen for five years and that was hard, though at least I'm alive, I guess, and who knows if Tamoxifen helped or not. My scars have tightened recently and I'm suffering pain down my arm, and my back is bad. I was referred to a physiotherapist by my GP. I had to wait ages, but she's helped by working into the scars and easing off the fascial restriction I had due to the scarring. I hadn't heard of fascia before. It's a layer of fibrous tissue that surrounds muscles, blood vessels and nerves. She can't cure me, though. They tighten up again quite quickly and stretching just causes me more problems. The physio has explained that because there are fascial connections throughout my body, it's not surprising my right hip gets so stiff and, as she's working on me, she's able to tell where it's pulling from, and it's usually the scars. I've started getting trapped nerves, again because of my scars – the nerves get trapped in tight tissue. This makes me feel ill, upsets my stomach and affects my ability to work. It's really horrible. Nobody seems to get that the effects of treatment can get worse over time. I wish they would – perhaps there'd be more support out there for us. I know I'm not alone with this, either. Someone said to me, not long ago, that I should stop moaning about my problems because her friend had just died of breast cancer and I should think myself lucky. I couldn't reply. I just cried, but I felt like saying 'That's terrible, I'm so sorry about your friend. The fact is though that the quality of my life is so rubbish that I often question whether it's worth living, no matter what you think.

If you can identify with Ruby's situation, whether to a greater or lesser extent, please do tell your GP how you're struggling. Equally, when you see your oncologist, please tell him or her and the breast care nurses. This way, perhaps there will in time be greater recognition of this problem, and **speaking openly about it may help you as well**, if you are affected in this way. Not everyone suffers as Ruby does, but the long-term effects of treatment are real and more widespread than we would imagine. If you are suffering, be assured that you are not alone!

Further reading

If you would like to read more about the issues raised in this book, my book on the psychological impact of breast cancer might be of interest to you. It also includes chapters on important subjects, such as working through breast cancer, that I have not been able to cover here.

Galgut C. *The Psychological Impact of Breast Cancer: a psychologist's insights as a patient.* Oxford: Radcliffe Publishing; 2010.

Finally

I wrote this poem a few years ago. Many women have read it and responded with 'That's it, that's how it is.' What do you think? Women have added their own words to my poem, too. Please feel free to do likewise. They have also used it to help them get through to people what it's really like having breast cancer.

Please don't …

Please don't tell me how I should feel
Or what I should think about having breast cancer;
How I should be 'over it' by now;
How I should be more positive;
How I should be grateful that I'm alive.

And please don't say, 'You're over-reacting to your situation,
It's only you who feels like this', or
'It's time you got on with your life.'

How can you know? *You* have never been in my situation.

And please don't ask me what I have contributed to my cancer
Or tell me how brave I've been.
There was no choice is all.
It was just the luck of the draw.

And please don't ask me how my breast cancer journey has been.
There *was* no journey.
There *is* no journey, because there is *no end in sight.*

And for pity's sake, don't say,
'Well, we're all going to die in the end,
I could get run over by a bus tomorrow.'

It's different.

You have never stared death head on.

You have never had breast cancer.
We are on different sides of the track now.

Tell me instead
That you cannot know what it is like living through this hell.

Tell me instead that you have an open heart
And an open mind,
That you'll listen,
That you'll try and understand,
Even when what I'm saying sounds preposterous to you.
It is my reality.

And please, please try and look beyond your own fears,
Or if you can't, tell me so.

Having breast cancer *is* terrifying
And the terror does *not* diminish,
Because the fear that it will come back *is* ever present.

So, please, please don't tell me that I'm one of the lucky ones,
That I'll be back to normal soon,

Because my *life* and *I* have been changed forever.

Just diagnosed

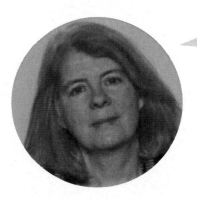

I'm so sorry you have just been diagnosed with breast cancer. Nobody wants this diagnosis. It's a truly horrible time for you and you are bound to be feeling incredibly upset, panicky, terrified, or maybe numb or a mixture of feelings. I know this because I was diagnosed twice myself in 2004, aged 49. I am also a counselling psychologist so am in a good position to offer you emotional support at this time.

No matter what your diagnosis, the good news is that these days most of us **live for years** after breast cancer, no matter whether we have primary or secondary breast cancer. However, it will very likely be hard, if not impossible, for you to hang on to this fact just now. Nevertheless, keep reminding yourself that this is so, as often as you can, and it might help to get you through the dark hours. Most of us think we are going to die, in the immediate aftermath of a diagnosis and for a good while afterwards, no matter how encouraging our doctors and nurses are. This is a perfectly normal psychological reaction to this news, and to be expected. Perhaps you're trying to keep control of yourself as much as possible at the moment, because you know you've got surgery coming up. Maybe you're keeping it together for your children, your partner, your friends or to hold down your job.

Photograph by kind permission of Macmillan Cancer Support

Remember that breast cancer is seldom a death sentence these days.

It's important to remember at this time that there is no right way to deal with breast cancer, now or later on. It might be a good idea just to go with what feels right for you, at this time, whilst you are digesting what is happening to you.

Shock

Perhaps you'll find that you relate to some of what Rumi says.

> *I was diagnosed a week ago now. I can't really think. I'm walking around like a zombie, trying to get my head around everything that has happened. I know I've got to have time off work, so I'm just concentrating on trying to get organised for that and worrying about the kids. I feel so bad for them that their Mum has breast cancer. I've got to be okay for them. I'm not sure how I'm going to get through all this, and I still can't really compute breast cancer and me having it. It feels completely surreal. I feel as though I'm in a bit of a bubble right now, watching people from afar. I can almost see myself going about my business, but it's as if I'm removed from everything. I hate feeling like this – sometimes it's more intense than others. Physically, I feel fine. It's so weird. How can I have cancer? There's no breast cancer in my family either. Is it my fault? I do all the right things to keep myself healthy, but that obviously hasn't worked.*

Rumi is in stunned shock. It is probably worth recognising at this point that you are, too. Some of us fall apart at this time, some of us semi-fall apart, but carry on anyway, and some of us react by feeling almost unaffected and, if asked, will say that we're fine. All of these reactions are just normal ways of coping. Try not to put extra pressure on yourself to feel anything you don't already feel. You have enough to cope with right now.

Our emotional responses are deep and cannot be easily controlled. That's just the way we are wired as human beings. Don't be surprised if you're experiencing lots of physical symptoms at the moment as well. Our emotions trigger physical responses in our bodies that can cause a range of sensations (e.g. gut disturbance, tight muscles, panic responses, itching, feeling very cold, etc.). Unpleasant though these are, they are perfectly normal and are unlikely to be a sign that your cancer is growing faster or spreading.

This was Rosa's response to realising that she might have breast cancer and then having it confirmed. Her reactions are very normal, and you might be able to relate to some of them:

Although it is six months ago now, I still remember all of the shocks of the diagnosis of breast cancer. When I felt a lump I couldn't believe there really was a lump there. When I went to the GP I couldn't believe she could feel that there really was a lump there.

At the breast clinic when the doctor who was doing the ultrasound said, 'I can see here what you are feeling,' that was the first indication I had that the lump I had felt might not be harmless. The temperature in the room seemed to drop, and the atmosphere in the room seemed to change. Even though I still didn't know, that was the first time I really felt that this could be serious.

When I then met the consultant and was told that it was 'suspicious' I just didn't know what to think. At that point I felt sure it was cancer, but nobody was saying it was cancer, they had to await the biopsy result for that.

When I went back for the result of the biopsy the consultant pulled his chair around the desk to sit next to me. 'The result shows that there is an abnormal growth, and it is cancer', he said. I couldn't hear any more after that. I just started shivering inside me, although outwardly I was calm. I felt nothing except the shock and the cold.

The sense of shock was so profound that there were no other conscious feelings. Just severe, sustained shock. I was numb. I couldn't believe that this was really happening. This could not be happening to me. I could not absorb it, I could not believe it.

Don't worry if you haven't reacted like Rosa. Some of us feel relatively fine and are not aware we are in shock. This is normal, too.

It's not your fault

Try not to give yourself a hard time about what you did or didn't do. Although there are known risk factors for developing breast cancer, even if we had them at diagnosis, this does not mean that they or we definitely caused our own breast cancer.

Remember that many women with the same risk factors or other ones haven't developed breast cancer, so **no one really knows with absolute certainty what causes this disease**. There is nothing wrong with giving something up if you feel it is necessary, at diagnosis or as time goes by, and it might make a difference and could help you feel that you have taken some control. However, whether you change your lifestyle or not is for you – and no one else – to decide. Overall, though, it is sometimes difficult for others to understand that a diagnosis of breast cancer is hard enough in itself, without adding guilt and blame to the equation.

Talking to doctors and nurses about your diagnosis and surgery

Many of us have questions we need to ask at diagnosis, and many of us feel awkward asking those in charge of our care and are not up to it at this time. Also, some of us don't have many questions at this stage. We just want the cancer out of us fast. Some of us will also have easier access to our cancer doctors and nurses than others.

However, each one of us has a right to ask questions and get answers, so that we can make the best decisions for ourselves at this time. It'll probably be hard for you to concentrate at present, and although some women want to keep their diagnosis to themselves, most of us want a close person with us at appointments, not least of all to ask questions and take notes.

Louise says:

Take someone with you to all appointments. There is nothing worse than being taken into those small consulting rooms to be told something awful and being alone. Of course, after the initial diagnosis, hopefully most of us won't be told something so horrible again, but still, it's worth having someone with you, even for check-ups.

Doctors and nurses are seldom trained in psychology. Some will understand the impact of the fact that you are in shock and want to consider your feelings, but others won't. If your doctor or nurse does not appear to understand, just say something like 'I'm sorry, but will you repeat that please? My concentration isn't good, because of the shock of the diagnosis.'

The reality is that even oncologists and specialist nurses, who work with women with breast cancer all the time, can only understand how you're feeling up to a point, unless they have been diagnosed themselves, but most of them will try to understand. If you feel strong enough, you can help them to understand by telling them how you feel, unless they appear unreceptive.

Remember that you have a right to say that you're not comfortable with decisions that are being made on your behalf, and to say no. Once the details of your surgery have been decided, you have a right to information about them and to ask questions, whether you are an NHS patient or a private one. This is your life and your body.

If you don't feel up to asking yourself, ask someone else, whom you trust, to help you out. Breast care nurses can be very helpful at this time. Their job is to be there for you at diagnosis and through your treatments, so your breast care nurse should be someone you can lean on.

Reactions of those around us

Most of us find that we don't have the energy to cope with others' reactions to our diagnosis, much as we might feel we should, and try to do so. Not everyone's reaction will be what we would like, either. If there is one time in your life when it's okay to be self-focused, it's surely now, even around your children, although I know how hard that is to put into practice, especially at this point. Also, some of us would rather focus on others at this time to help us get through, and that's okay, too. Just remember, though, that being in shock saps energy, as does worrying about the future.

If you have people around you in your personal life whom you can lean on, this is the time to do so and ask them for help, if you feel able to. Most of us find that not everyone we would have imagined would be there for us will be. Sometimes it is the people who are normally less involved with us who are able to support us better than those closer to us. Also, people can surprise us in a good way at this time. At the moment, if you can, it might be best for you to try not to worry about the people who aren't there for you.

The following is an example of how a newly diagnosed woman called Mary felt a week after being diagnosed. Perhaps you will identify with some of what she says:

> *I was diagnosed with breast cancer last week. I know I have to have surgery as soon as there is a bed available, but I don't have a date yet. I'm also not totally sure what kind of cancer I've got or how advanced it is. I couldn't really follow what the doctor said to me. I can't say I really feel anything much right now, except that I feel sick all the time and I keep thinking I'm going to die. I've told my husband, but it's like I'm looking at him through a glass wall. I don't think he knows how to be with me, but I know he's really upset and frantic, too. It feels as though my whole world is falling apart and I can't stop it happening.*

As a counselling psychologist, the first thing I would say to Mary is that her reaction is totally normal. A lot of us will not follow everything our doctors tell us at this time, and get lost in it all. We're only human and we're in extreme shock. When Mary says that she feels as if she's looking at her husband through a glass wall, it is shock that is making her feel like this – almost removed from the situation as though she's watching things happening from a distance.

It might help Mary to get more information about her breast cancer from her doctor – either from the doctor who diagnosed her, if she can contact them, or by asking her GP to find out more for her. She could also contact a breast care nurse for further information. This might help her to feel a little less frightened. Some people want more information than others at this point, but Mary has a right to expect an appointment with her surgeon, or someone in their team, to explain what kind of surgery they are recommending and give her a choice about which kind of surgery she has. It might be best for her to take a friend, who is able to listen and take things in, with her to this appointment and arrange that appointment if she's not up to organising it herself. There should also be a breast care nurse available to help Mary out.

It's very hard for Mary, knowing that her husband is so upset, but not feeling able to connect with him. However, many of us, like Mary, cannot support those close to us at this time. We need all our energy for us. Sometimes it is enough to say to the people around us 'Look, it's an awful time at the moment. We're just going to have to get through it as best we can.' Sometimes letting them know that we're not up to taking on their feelings can help. Also, saying it's okay for them to talk to friends or the professionals can help during such an immensely difficult time, because it gives them an outlet, thereby taking some pressure off us.

It can be helpful to get some emotional support from a trained counsellor whilst waiting for surgery, but we don't all have access to one. The role of a counsellor at this point would be to understand your situation as best they can and to support you by talking about whatever you want to raise, without judging you. You would be encouraged to be as easy on yourself as you can be.

If you do not have a counsellor available to you face to face, or even if you do, organisations such as Breast Cancer Care and Macmillan Cancer Support have helplines you can phone for support and Internet forums you can join:

Breast Cancer Care   www.breastcancercare.org.uk
Helpline 0808 800 6000

Macmillan Cancer Support   www.macmillan.org.uk
Helpline 0808 808 0000

The Haven Breast Cancer Support Centres (www.thehaven.org.uk) in London, Hereford and Leeds offer a wide range of face to face support.

London   020 7384 0099

Hereford   01432 361061

Leeds   01132 847829

Louise found the Breast Cancer Care buddy scheme helpful:

I found it really helpful to have a 'cancer buddy.' Breast Cancer Care runs a scheme. My buddy was about six years post-treatment. She was similar to me in terms of age, family, type of cancer, genetic link and treatment. She was great during my treatment, would call me every couple of weeks for a chat. I really felt I could say anything to her.

Telling people

Soon after being diagnosed, some of us want to tell everyone about our diagnosis, and feel better for doing so. Others tell only a few people, and some keep their diagnosis to themselves. It can be hard to know how to handle work colleagues, but this is a matter of individual choice at this time. Sometimes the hardest thing is telling those we love, as Sarah found out:

Telling people was one of the things I found most difficult after diagnosis. I felt like I was continually making the people I cared about most in the world cry. I avoided seeing some people because I couldn't take dealing with their worry and sadness when I didn't know how to deal with it myself. I found it helpful to tell my immediate circle of close friends, then asked them to tell other friends when they felt it appropriate. This felt a lot easier on everyone as people had time to adjust to their own feelings before they contacted me.

This was what happened when Louise told her son:

I didn't tell my son for a few days and didn't really eat until I had. Once I told him (he was 11), I suddenly felt really hungry for the first time in ages. He asked me if I would die. I said I really hoped not. Then we talked about what his dad would let him do that I don't if I did die (eat pizza, not wear his bicycle helmet, not having to tidy his room). It sounds weird but it actually helped.

Whom we tell and how we tell them is for us – and no one else – to decide. There is no right way to behave at this time, either. It might be a good idea to keep reminding yourself that **there is no right way to handle a diagnosis of breast cancer**. There is also no right way to cope with surgery or the treatments. This will help to support you during the coming months.

After surgery

After surgery, your doctors will be in a better position to decide which additional treatments you will need. Again, you have a right to as much information as you want about the options available. Ultimately, it is your choice whether you go ahead with them, but most women choose to.

This can be an incredibly confusing time. You will be tired and overawed from surgery, so this is a time to involve others, if you can. Your breast care nurse can help you, too. Some women want more information about their treatments than others, but many women find that being told what to expect helps them through. They can be more of a shock if you're not prepared for them. Equally, if you prepare for the worst, it is possible to find one or more of the treatments easier than you had feared.

A final reminder

There have been huge advances in the treatment of breast cancer. Breast cancer is no longer seen as the killer disease it used to be. In fact, these days it is increasingly viewed as a chronic condition. Keep reminding yourself of this. It may well help you get through.

References

1   Murray J. Okay, I thought – cope with it. *The Guardian*, 2 October 2008.

2   Galgut C. *The Psychological Impact of Breast Cancer, a psychologist's insights as a patient.* Oxford: Radcliffe Publishing; 2010. p. 59.

3   Galgut C, op. cit., p. 119.

4   Coyne JC, Pajak TF, Harris J et al. Emotional well-being does not predict survival in head and neck cancer patients. *Cancer.* 2007; 110: 2568–75.

5   Galgut C, op. cit., p. 101.

6   Bakewell J. *The View From Here: life at seventy.* London: Atlantic Books; 2006. p. 227.

7   Macmillan Cancer Support. *Cured – but at what cost?* Macmillan, July 2013.